Acknowledgement

Special thanks to my wonderful husband, Ron, for his unconditional love and support. I could not have done this without you.

I would also like to thank Dr. Zach LaBoube and Debbie O'Phelan for their contributions, not only to the book, but to dieters everywhere.

Thank you for reading. If you enjoy this book, please leave a review at the website where you purchased the book.

All rights reserved. Aside from brief quotations for media coverage and reviews, no part of this book may be reproduced or distributed in any form without the author's permission.

Thank you for supporting authors and a diverse, creative culture by purchasing this book and complying with copyright laws.

Copyright © 2017 by Lara Plogman

Interior design by Pronoun

Beta reading by Ron Plogman

Proof reading by William Johns

ISBN: 9781537894454

Table of Contents

Acknowledgement 1

Disclaimer 7

Chapter 1 - Welcome 9

Chapter 2 - Dr. ATW Simeons 13

Chapter 3 - Studies On hCG 15

Chapter 4 - Effects Of hCG On The Body 17

Chapter 5 - Sugar Addiction 21

Chapter 6 - Ketosis 25

Chapter 7 - What Kind Of Results Can You Expect? 31

Chapter 8 - Duration Of hCG Treatment 33

Chapter 9 - Protocol Comparisons 35

Chapter 10 - Original Protocol 39

Chapter 11 - 2.0 Protocol 41

Chapter 12 - 3.0 Protocol 47

Chapter 13 - Rogue Dieters 53

Chapter 14 - Intermittent Fasting 55

Chapter 15 - Before Photos And Measurements 57

Chapter 16 - Phase One Loading 59

Chapter 17 - Meal Prep 63

Chapter 18 - Traveling And Eating Out 65

Chapter 19 - Protein Shakes, Green Smoothies And Juicing 69

Chapter 20 - Hunger 71

Chapter 21 - Alcohol 73

Chapter 22 - Stalls 75

Chapter 23 - Dieting Tools 81

Chapter 24 - Phase 3 And Maintenance 83

Chapter 25 - Time Between Rounds..87

Chapter 26 - Naysayers And Critics 89

Chapter 27 - Choosing Which Form Of hCG To Use 91

Chapter 28 - Choosing A Start Date 97

Chapter 29 - Missed Doses...99

Chapter 30 - Cheat Days...101

Chapter 31 - In Conclusion...103

Glossary..105

Disclaimer

The publisher and author are not responsible for any specific health or allergy needs that may require medical supervision and are not liable for any damages or negative consequences from any treatment, action, application or preparation, to any person reading or following the information in this book.

The information in this book has not been evaluated by the Food and Drug Administration.

I am not, nor am I holding myself out to be a doctor/physician, nurse, physician's assistant, advanced practice nurse, or any other medical professional ("Medical Provider"), psychiatrist, psychologist, therapist, counselor, or social worker ("Mental Health Provider"), registered dietician or licensed nutritionist, or member of the clergy. As a wellness coach, I am not providing health care, medical or nutritional therapy services, or attempting to diagnose, treat, prevent or cure any physical, mental or emotional issue, disease or condition.

The information provided in or through this book pertaining to your health and wellness, or any other aspect of your life is not intended to be a substitute for the professional medical advice, diagnosis or treatment provided by your own medical provider or mental health provider.

You agree and acknowledge that I am not providing medical advice, mental health advice, or religious advice in any way. Always seek the advice of your own medical provider and/or mental health provider regarding any questions or concerns you have about your specific health or any medications, herbs or supplements you are currently taking and before implementing any recommendations or suggestions from this book. Do not disregard medical advice or delay seeking medical advice because of information you have read in this book.

Do not start or stop taking any medications without speaking to your own medical provider or mental health provider. If you have or suspect that you have a medical or mental health problem, contact your own medical provider or mental health provider promptly.

My role as the author is to support and assist you in reaching your own goals, but your success depends primarily on your own effort, motivation, commitment and follow-through. I cannot predict and I do not guarantee that you will attain a particular result, and you accept and understand that results differ for each individual. Each individual's results depend on his or her unique background, dedication, desire, motivation, actions, and numerous other factors. You fully agree that there are no guarantees as to the specific outcome or results you can expect from using the information you receive in this book.

Any recommendations for what or when to eat are strictly listed as discussion points to help jumpstart your conversation with your physician or licensed dietician, and not be construed as medical advice.

References are provided for informational purposes only and do not constitute endorsement of any websites or other sources. Readers should be aware that the websites listed in this book may change.

Chapter 1 - Welcome

You've heard the warning from friends and family that hCG doesn't work, and that a low-calorie diet does more harm than good. But you've also seen the numerous before and after photos and success stories from the people who have tried the hCG diet, so obviously, something is working. So, what do you do?

Let me start by saying probably the most important thing first. **hCG does not cause you to lose weight. However, hCG will work as a natural appetite suppressant while you do a very low calorie diet. The diet is what will cause the weight loss, not the hCG.**

Are you with me so far? It is extremely important that you know this right off the bat. hCG is not a miracle cure for obesity. But it is very effective in controlling your appetite when used properly while you eat a low-calorie diet, and it doesn't have those terrible side effects that you get when you consume most pharmaceuticals for appetite control.

Dr. Simeons wrote in the American Journal of Clinical Nutrition, September 1963. "What so many investigators seem to overlook is that human chorionic gonadotrophin (hCG) as such has no weight-reducing action whatsoever, nor has this ever been claimed to be the case. In fact, those quite exceptional patients who have the willpower to stay on a 500-calorie diet for forty days without human chorionic gonadotrophin often lose more weight than those who are receiving it; but they look drawn and haggard and regain their weight rapidly as soon as they stop dieting, because they have depleted normal fat reserves.

The function of human chorionic gonadotrophin is exclusively to make drastic reduction over a short period of time safe, comfortable and entirely confined to abnormal fat deposits. It is the latter peculiarity which accounts for the relative ease with which patients can hold their weight after this treatment."

Pharmaceutical appetite suppressants such as benzphetamine, diethylpropion, mazindol and phentermine have a long list of reported side effects that include:

- Increased heart rate
- Increased blood pressure
- Sweating
- Constipation
- Insomnia
- Excessive thirst
- Lightheadedness
- Drowsiness

I'm assuming that if you have purchased this book, you have already made the decision that you want to try the hCG diet and are wanting to learn the best way to go about it. So here is the part where I remind you that I'm not a doctor, but a well experienced dieter and wellness coach who has done much research over the years. Most importantly, I get to remind that you should consult with your physician before beginning the hCG diet or any other diet, and keep your physician aware of complications that you become aware of during the diet.

If your physician tells you that you have a medical condition that would prevent you from doing this diet, please take their advice and choose a different diet, or find a healthy way to modify the diet that your physician is agreeable to.

In this book, I want to discuss the original protocol developed by Dr. ATW Simeons in *Pounds and Inches*, and discuss some of the newer protocols including rogue protocols so you can make an informed decision before beginning the diet. You may even choose to switch protocols during a round just to test the waters to see if your body responds better to one protocol than the other or to break a stall.

For those of you who are new to the hCG diet, I will discuss terms that we use during the diet as they come up, and I will include a glossary at the end of the book for your reference. For the many of you who have done the original protocol diet in the past but are looking for new options, please hang in there while we discuss some of the basics and then start with the original protocol.

Chapter 2 - Dr. ATW Simeons

Dr. ATW Simeons was the British endocrinologist who developed the hCG diet. It is helpful to know more about the credibility of the man who has helped so many of us achieve our weight loss goals.

Dr. Simeons was born in 1900 in London, and he died in 1970 in Rome. Before his work with hCG, Dr. Simeons was awarded the Red Cross Order of Merit for his groundbreaking work with malaria, and conducted extensive studies on the bubonic plague and leprosy in India. While working with malnourished women in India, he noticed that despite the mother's malnutrition, they were delivering healthy babies.

He shifted his focus to weight loss and obesity in the 1950's while in Rome. He began giving hCG to young boys suffering from Froehlich Syndrome. These boys were considered "fat" and had oversized breasts and undersized sexual organs. Dr. Simeons noticed that the hCG was helping the boys lose their hunger and inches around their hips.

That's when a woman came to visit him in his clinic and ask for his help. He noticed that even though she looked thin and drawn in the upper body, she was obese from the hips down. Dr. Simeons began treating the woman with 125 IU's of hCG with daily injections. She lost eight inches in her hips in only eight weeks. He claimed that by combining a calorie-restrictive diet with hCG and 30 minutes of low intensity exercise the woman could rid herself of stored fat.

In the late 1960s Dr. Simeon's clinic in Rome was treating the rich and famous from around the world for obesity. He wrote *Pounds And Inches: A New Approach To Obesity* to help him educate other doctors and hospitals about the hCG diet. In it he claims that men and women who used his diet found relief from headaches, hunger pain, irritability and fatigue by using hCG with their diet. If you would like to read *Pounds And Inches*, you can download a copy for free on our website at www.MyHCGWellness.net.

Many healthcare professionals still prescribe hCG for weight loss even though it is not approved by the FDA for that purpose. This is called "off-label" use. But many dieters are still having great success with the diet today with hCG. One of the biggest concerns will always be how a very low calorie diet, such as the 500 calories per day diet affects the body.

Each person is different, and their bodies will react differently. That is one of the main reasons doctors are recommending a low-calorie diet (800-1000 calories per day) rather than the very low calorie diet. This is a decision that should be made by you and a physician who knows your medical history and can monitor your progress.

Chapter 3 - Studies On hCG

Your body is designed to store fat to convert to energy in times when it has no food. Many people who promote the hCG diet will try to convince you that using hCG will cause your body to target the fat stores in your body rather than targeting muscle. There have been numerous studies on this theory including *Craig (1963), Ashley/Harper (1973), Stein (1976), Young (1976), Sheety (1977), Greenway (1977), Birmingham (1983), Lijeson (1995), and Emma (2012)*. The findings have been mixed on whether less muscle is lost with hCG, but the studies have not been consistent across the board in the way they were conducted, including on which parts of the body the measurements were taken.

The President of the American Society of Bariatric Physicians performed a six-week study in 2010 on a modified 800 calorie hCG diet using sublingual (placed under the tongue) hCG. They compared 19 hCG patients to 19 people without hCG using an 800 calorie per day diet. The results? The dieters on hCG lost an average of 19.84 pounds in the six weeks. The dieters who did not use hCG lost an average of 14.75 pounds. The BMI (Body Mass Index) of the hCG group decreased by 3.18, and the non-hCG group decreased their BMI by 2.48. Their conclusion was, "Sublingual hCG appeared to be significantly better in weight loss than a similar meal replacement diet of comparable protein and calorie composition.

The results revealed a relatively rapid weight loss in six weeks with preservation of lean body mass. Furthermore, it appears that this approach could have a benefit to the patients in that they demonstrated reduced usage of controlled substances for appetite." You can read further about this study at the American Journal of Clinical Nutrition's website at www.ajcn.org or at the American Society of Bariatric Physicians Research in their study "Effect of human chorionic gonadotrophin on weight loss, hunger and feeling of well-being" authored by W.L. Asher, MD and Harold W. Harper, MD.

The American Journal of Clinical Nutrition reported in Volume 26, 211-218, copyright 1973, the following: Twenty female patients on 500 to 550 calorie diets receiving daily injections of 125 IU of hCG were compared to 20 female patients on 500 to 550 calorie diets receiving placebo injections. Patients were instructed to return for daily injections six days per week for a total of 36 injections. The hCG group lost significantly more mean weight, had a significantly greater mean weight loss per injection, and lost a significantly greater mean percentage of their starting weight. The percentage of affirmative daily patient responses indicating little or no hunger and feeling good to excellent was significantly greater in the hCG group than in the placebo group.

All of these tests only focused on obese women rather than men or women who were overweight but not obese. Seven of the nine studies concluded there was no difference in muscle loss, while two studies claimed there was less muscle loss with the hCG dieters.

It may be interesting to note that the most recent study claims there was less muscle loss, whereas the other studies were much older. So perhaps the foods in our modern diet affect the amount of fat to muscle ratio. Hopefully we will see more modern and consistent tests in the near future.

Because there was not much consistency in conducting the tests or the way in which results were recorded, it is hard to give a definite answer on whether you lose more fat than muscle with hCG.

The same can be said about whether a dieter can lose more weight overall with hCG. Since the majority of the studies showed little difference in the amount of weight lost with dieters taking hCG and dieters receiving placebo, I cannot assume that hCG does promote weight loss in any other way than by helping control appetite. But on a more positive note, we can assume that hCG does not hinder weight loss during dieting.

Chapter 4 - Effects Of hCG On The Body

Let me start this chapter by reminding you to review the disclaimer at the beginning of this book and reminding you that I am not a doctor. Your overall health is far more important than losing weight, so always check with your physician about any symptoms and keep your doctor informed of changes so that her or she can properly monitor your progress and offer their advice.

When using the correct dosage of hCG, which is a minimal amount, there is no evidence that hCG is dangerous. While hCG has not been approved by the FDA for weight loss treatments, it has been approved in much larger dosages for other medical treatments including treating infertility in women and increasing sperm count in men. But as dieters we are focused only on the minimal dosage which will curb your hunger and cravings during the diet.

Interestingly enough, when taking hCG to control appetite you would decrease the dosage if you are still experiencing hunger rather than increase the dosage. The goal should always be to take the minimal dose possible.

If you are taking the injections for hCG, you may experience some mild redness and swelling at the injection site. There may even be some small bruising. If this is bothersome to you, make sure you check some of the many videos online about how to correctly inject yourself or try injecting into a different area of the body.

During the first week using hCG you may experience headaches. The most common cause of a headache is dehydration, but if you know you are adequately hydrated, the headaches could be caused from "keto flu" or your body adjusting to ketosis and withdrawing from sugar and carbohydrates, and possibly even caffeine withdrawal depending on the foods you have chosen to eliminate. The medications you normally take to alleviate headaches should not cause any drug interactions with the hCG. The headaches should only last for a few days while your body is adjusting. Try to think of the headaches as a detoxing of your body. Obviously, if something about the headaches feels unusual to you or they last longer than ten days, please see your doctor as you may have other medical conditions going on.

If you experience issues such as upset stomach, diarrhea or constipation, those could be signs of food allergies or your body adjusting to eating different foods. Again, over the counter medications that you would normally take to alleviate symptoms should not have any drug interaction with the hCG, but it is always best to check with your physician. However, if you notice that the symptoms only occur when you eat a specific food, then you should consider that the issue is caused from a food allergy and possibly eliminating that food from your diet permanently.

Once you begin the low-calorie portion of the diet, you may notice a decreased number of bowel movements. This is normal because you are putting less junk in your body and adding more healthy foods that your body is absorbing and using. Of course, if you are uncomfortable or feel like you are becoming constipated, a suppository should bring quick relief. You may also want to consider adding additional fiber to your diet in the form of psyllium capsules, but add them gradually and increase your water intake.

Dizziness is uncommon, but it could happen while your body is adjusting to the lower calories. It could also happen if you are dehydrated. Stay hydrated!

A more rare side effect of the diet, not the hCG, is leg or muscle cramps. This is normally caused by a lack of potassium and is easily remedied with potassium supplements as recommended by your doctor.

If you should develop a rash soon after starting the low-calorie phase, this is possible caused from your body releasing toxins that have built up in your body over years of poor eating habits. Again, your typical ointments or creams are often used to treat the rash, as well as a little coconut oil to help relieve itching and irritation. If this symptom lasts more than ten days, you should consult your physician.

I would never suggest giving hCG to a child for weight loss without consulting a physician and having them monitor the progress. When used with young boys, hCG may cause early onset of puberty.

On the original protocol, Dr. Simeons recommended that you discontinue any prescription medications and supplements other than coral calcium. Obviously, discontinuing prescription medications is not a good idea without consulting your physician. We will discuss the various protocols later in this book, but with the hCG 2.0 and 3.0 diets, prescription meds and supplements are still allowed. Even fish oil/Omega 3 supplements. Dr. LaBoube, author of *HCG 2.0,* also recommends taking a multivitamin, biotin, and potassium supplements. I have seen other doctors recommend adding a fat burner/calcium pyruvate and probiotics. Again, please consult your physician when necessary before adding supplements to your diet. The supplements are not as important on your loading days as they will be in phase two. They are not required for phase two, but they may ease any side effects from the low-calorie phase.

Chapter 5 - Sugar Addiction

Phase two of the hCG diet is the perfect opportunity to break a sugar addiction you may not have even known you had. Let's briefly discuss how kicking refined sugar from your diet helps your body just after the first week.

1. You could see a 10% decrease in LDL cholesterol and a 20 to 30% decrease in triglycerides which should make your heart happy.
2. Sugar is a food that can cause inflammation, so anyone suffering from adult acne could be seeing a noticeable difference in their complexion.
3. A Columbia University study found that women who eat a diet high in added sugars and refined grains are more likely to experience anxiety, irritability and mood swings. Many women start to notice more of a feeling of well-being at this point.
4. Sugar triggers the body's release of cortisol which can interfere with your sleep cycles. Breaking the sugar addiction can have you waking up feeling more refreshed and with more energy.

The average person consumes up to 15 teaspoons per day of sugar without even realizing it because it is hidden in so much processed foods. Even foods you wouldn't necessarily think about such as sauces, yogurts and protein shakes. In fact, sugar in one form or another is in 74% of packaged foods. Does that shock you? It should.

The American Heart Association recommends no more than 9 teaspoons (38 grams) of sugar per day for men, and six teaspoons (25 grams) per day for women.

Common names for sugar on food packaging include:
- Sugar
- Sucrose
- High Fructose Corn Syrup
- Agave Nectar
- Molasses
- Cane Juice
- Carob Syrup
- Fruit Juice
- Honey
- Golden Syrup
- Sorghum Syrup
- Barley Malt
- Corn Syrup
- Dextrin
- Dextrose
- Glucose
- Ethyl Maltol
- Fructose

As you can see, the list is not an easy one for most of us to remember. And food manufacturers do not want you to remember them. Sugar makes their food taste good, and keeps consumers wanting more.

Be wary of anything that says, "No added sugar", "Made with real fruit", or "Made with whole grains", or "No high-fructose corn syrup". Many of those items will still contain sugar in some form. Get into the habit of reading ingredients and nutritional values on every packaged food you purchase.

Once you cut sugar from your diet, you may well never want to re-introduce it. I was on a very low sugar diet before beginning the hCG diet, but now I am even more cautious about eating it. There is so much hidden sugar in the foods we eat. If I get too much sugar now I almost immediately get a headache, and that is usually followed by stomach pains. I try now to reserve sugar for special events, such a bite of birthday cake, or a bite of Christmas candy.

But no more whole slices of cake or full size candy bars. It's not worth the headache.

There is a great documentary called *That Sugar Film* (2014) that looks at the hidden dangers in sugar and its effect on the body. It's very eye-opening and will have you wanting to ban sugar in your life forever.

Chapter 6 - Ketosis

I want to spend a little extra time on this section because ketosis is so important to success with the hCG diet. It is also the way of eating that most dieters choose to adopt in phase three (between rounds) and phase four (maintaining your weight after you have reached your goal weight).

Ketosis is a normal state for your body to be in while fasting or on a low carb diet. It involves a considerable reduction in carbohydrate intake, and an increase of fat intake. The reduced carb intake puts your body into a metabolic state called ketosis, which many people automatically relate to the Atkins Diet. However, hCG diets are not high protein diets. Eating high protein can affect your insulin levels, and many doctors claim that this can stall your weight loss.

The "keto" in the word ketosis derives from the process of when the body produces small fuel molecules called ketones. Ketones are produced in the liver and are an alternative fuel for the body, used when blood sugar (glucose) is in short supply. And best of all, this causes your body to burn fat at a much higher rate.

The Journal of Clinical Endocrinology and Metabolism published the results of a six-month study in April of 2003 that concluded, "The very low carbohydrate diet group lost more weight (8.5 +/- 1.0 vs. 3.9 +/- 1.0 kg; $P < 0.001$) and more body fat (4.8 +/- 0.67 vs. 2.0 +/- 0.75 kg; $P < 0.01$) than the low-fat diet group. Mean levels of blood pressure, lipids, fasting glucose, and insulin were within normal ranges in both groups at baseline.

Based on this data, a very low carbohydrate diet is more effective than a low-fat diet for short-term weight loss and, over six months, is not associated with deleterious effects on important cardiovascular risk factors in healthy women."

Diabetic Medicine: The Journal Of The British Diabetic Association reported in December of 2007 that weight loss was over three times greater on a low-carb diet than on a low-fat diet. That's a big difference.

The process of converting from glucose to ketones can take approximately two days or more, which is why the first few days of the diet can sometimes be challenging. Some of the side effects you may experience during this transformation are:

- Tiredness or fatigue
- Leg Cramps
- Headache
- Feeling thirsty all the time
- Bad breath
- Metallic taste in the mouth
- Weakness
- Dizziness
- Nausea or stomach ache
- Sleep problems

Compare that to the health benefits, such as reduced insulin and blood glucose levels (which is especially good for type 2 Diabetes and Prediabetes), improved symptoms for Parkinson's Disease, better skin complexion, reduction of seizures in epileptic children, slowed progression of Alzheimer's, slowed tumor growth in cancer patients, decreased levels of heart disease, and the issue we are focusing on right now, weight loss.

Usually, the only types of people who need to worry about ketosis are those people with type 1 diabetes, breastfeeding mothers with type 2 diabetes, and extreme athletes. In these circumstances, you should have your physician monitor your ketone levels to make sure they do not get too high, and that you are getting enough carbs in your diet.

The three main types of ketosis diet are:

1. Cyclical - Spending a set number of days in ketosis and then a set number of days out of ketosis. For example, you may spend seven days on a standard ketosis diet, but then drastically increase your carbs for two days, and repeat that process. This version is often used by athletes so they can increase their carbs on heavy workout days.

2. Standard - very low-carb, moderate-protein and high-fat diet. An example would be 75% fat, 20% protein and 5% carbs.

3. High-protein - similar to the standard diet, but with increased protein. This could look like 60% fat, 35% protein and 5% carbs.

In a normal ketosis diet you may find many foods that are low carb and high fat (LCHF for short). That type of diet is prohibited in the original protocol. The hCG original protocol diet is not considered a ketosis diet because it is not low carb.

You can monitor whether your body is in ketosis with Ketostix, which are available at most drugstores in the US for around $10. Some people prefer to monitor their ketosis levels while on the diet, but most of us do not worry about it as long as we are sticking to the diet plan.

Some of the signs that you are in ketosis are:

1. Bad breath. Once you reach full ketosis your elevated ketone levels will exit your body through your urine and through your breath. Sugarless chewing gum helps, and you can always keep a toothbrush with you. This will eventually go away with most people.

2. Increased focus and energy. When you are entering ketosis, you may feel a brain fog and tiredness. However, once you reach ketosis not only will those symptoms go away, your blood sugar will stabilize giving you more energy, and your

brain will start burning ketones instead of glucose which will help you focus for longer periods of time.

3. Short term decrease in physical performance. It takes your muscles a little longer to adjust to reduced glycogen levels, but this only lasts a few weeks. Your body will return to normal functioning levels once they adjust, and if you are in ketosis you can burn as much as 230% more fat with normal everyday activities such as walking if you stay in ketosis.

4. Increased urination. Ketones act as a diuretic.

5. Dry mouth as a result of the increased urination

Fat is the most calorie-dense of the three macronutrients, with 9 calories per gram. In the original protocol the claim is that If you eat excessive amounts of high-fat foods, you run the risk of gaining weight. The 3.0 protocol has a much highest fat consumption, so if you are struggling with giving up your fatty foods, then definitely consider starting with the 3.0 protocol.

So, what kind of foods should you avoid in a ketogenic diet? Anything with sugar or starch is a definite no-go. That includes things like fruit juices, candy, rice, bread, pasta or cereal. Beans and legumes are also out (such as peas, chickpeas, kidney beans) as well as root vegetables (such as potatoes, carrots, and parsnips).

You also need to be careful with anything marked sugar-free as these items often contain sugar alcohols. That is not to say that some things can be enjoyed in moderation if you are monitoring your carb intake.

When we discuss phase three and maintenance later we will go into more detail on what you can eat, but the things you do want to eat include, meats, poultry, fish, eggs, butter, cream, cheese, nuts, avocado, healthy fats and low-carb vegetables. Keep in mind that the original protocol and 2.0 protocol will limit some of these items while in the low-calorie phase (phase two).

Virtually every dieter that completes a round of the hCG diet and sticks to the protocol will lose a significant amount of weight. The diet is certainly one of the strictest in terms of its allowable foods and daily calorie requirements, but it's by far one of the most effective diets available anywhere.

Chapter 7 - What Kind Of Results Can You Expect?

This answer will of course vary by person. You will most commonly hear people and advertisements stating that women can expect to lose a half pound per day, and that men typically lose one pound per day. Those numbers tend to be consistent with what I have observed in most of my dieters, but this is not guaranteed.

Dieters who have much more weight to lose do tend to lose weight faster than those with only a few pounds to lose. It's not uncommon for me to see heavier dieters lose 2-3 pounds per day, especially in the first two weeks.

I also see some dieters that lose less than a half pound per day. This often happens when a dieter is closer to their goal weight.

Another big reason for varied results is that some dieters are continually looking for loopholes and want to push their carb and sugar intake. So, they tend to have lesser results. And of course, there are the dieters who cheat occasionally even though they deny it.

If you are closely monitoring the ingredients in your foods and staying within the guidelines, you should have good results. Attitude goes a long way with the hCG diet. So, to ensure your greatest successes, choose a plan and learn how to live comfortably within it rather than make excuses to eat whatever you want.

Chapter 8 - Duration Of hCG Treatment

The most common durations of phase two (the low-calorie phase) are 23-28 days (short round) and 40-56 days (long round.) That does not include the three days following your last dose while you are still on the low-calorie diet. That is just the number of days taking hCG. Dr. Simeons recommended doing phase two for a minimum of 23 days to achieve the desired effect on the hypothalamus gland and allow you to maintain your weight loss. However, many people, including myself, choose to do phase two for forty days at a time.

Short rounds are perfect for people who only wish to lose 10 or 15 pounds, or for people know they have an event coming up where they know they won't have a chance to stay on protocol, such as a big Thanksgiving gathering or vacation. Short rounds are also better for people who just have trouble maintaining their willpower for longer periods of time. Dr. Simeons advised his patients to continue to take their hCG a full 23 days even if they reached their goal weight before they finished, but to increase their calorie intake to 800-1000 for the remaining days on hCG.

The long rounds are great for people who dread the loading phase and know that they want to lose 20 pounds or more. Some people doing injections skip a dose one day a week which allows them to extend their duration to 47 days, but they are still only taking 40 days of injections. Dr. Simeons recommended not taking more than 40 days of hCG to avoid becoming immune to the hCG. I cannot say that there is evidence of becoming immune to hCG, but I can say that extending a very low or low calorie diet for any longer than 47 days should only be done with your doctor's consent and monitoring. You do not want to put any extra stress on your body. Moving into phase three you will be allowing your body to replenish itself and prepare itself for the next round if you choose to do one.

Fat burning is work, and your body needs to rest sometimes. That doesn't mean go back to carbs and sugar. That simply means adding more calories back into your diet while still making healthy food choices.

Keep in mind that you can start the diet with the intention of doing a long round, but if you need to stop due to illness or other unforeseen circumstance that you want to try to complete at least 21 days if you can before stopping unless you or your doctor feel it medically necessary to stop before then. Just because you start a round does not mean it is mandatory to finish. You will not do permanent damage to your metabolism if you stop a round early. Your overall health is far more important than losing weight with this diet. So, if at any time you feel you are unable to function in a healthy manner, or your physician advises you to stop the diet and hCG for medical reasons, please stop immediately.

Always wait the recommended time between rounds before starting a new round, and always fat load for two or three days at the start of each round.

Chapter 9 - Protocol Comparisons

	Original Protocol	2.0 Protocol	3.0 Protocol
	PROTOCOL COMPARISON CHART		
Loading Days	Fat load including high carbs foods & sugar	Recommend healthy fat loading, low carb & no sugar	Recommend high healthy fat loading, low carb & no sugar, starch, grain or gluten
Calorie Limit	500/day	40% of BMR, counting protein calories only, max. 1000/day	Calculated at 40% & 55% deficit of BMR
Carb Limit	Moderate carbs, but no set limit	30 grams/day	20 grams/day
Exercise	Not allowed	Allowed as dieter was doing before diet, encourages 30 min. walking before breakfast.	Encourages 30 min. exercise in fasted state, light weights may be added
Alcohol	In moderation	In moderation	In moderation, include in daily macros, dry red or white wine, liquor mixed with zero calorie mixers
Approved Food List	Yes	None	None

	PROTOCOL COMPARISON CHART Cont.		
	Original Protocol	**2.0 Protocol**	**3.0 Protocol**
Beverages	Limited to water, coffee, tea	Any zero calorie/zero carb drinks allowed	Any zero calorie/zero carb drinks allowed
Breakfast	Tea or coffee only	Encourages high protein, low calorie breakfast within 30 minutes of waking	Depends on intermittent fasting schedule
Dairy	None allowed	Allowed	Full fat including kefir and yogurt, counted in daily macros
Eating Before Bed	No info	Choose a lean protein source	Depends on intermittent fasting schedule
Fruits	Apples, strawberries, orange, grapefruit	None other than juice of one lemon or lime/day	None, but berries are ok for some people
Oil Lotion Cosmetics	Not allowed	No restrictions	No restrictions
Other Medications	None	As prescribed by your doctor	As prescribed by your doctor

	PROTOCOL COMPARISON GROUP Cont.		
	Original Protocol	**2.0 Protocol**	**3.0 Protocol**
Phase Three	No restrictions except starches and sugar for first 3 weeks	Daily calories 125% of BMR, 40% protein, 40% fats, 20% carbs, recommends carbs only come from fruit & root vegetables, rolling carb number to next day is ok	Cycling one day at full BMR, next day 20% BMR
Proteins	Restricted to beef, veal, chicken and white fish, lobster, crab, shrimp, unless vegetarian	No restrictions, but lean proteins encouraged	Depends on BMR & glucose, 60 to 100grams
Starches	Melba toast or Grissini bread	None	None
Supplements	Only calcium, vitamins C & D in non-oily format	No restrictions	Electrolytes, sole water (pink sea salt) magnesium, vitamin C & Smooth Move tea
Vegetables	Limited choices, no mixing	No restriction within daily carb limit, mixing is ok, not necessary to count calories	Non-starchy, mixing is ok

Chapter 10 - Original Protocol

Dr. Simeons Protocol for phase two can be summarized as follows:

- Calories limited to 500 per day
- Only tea or black coffee for breakfast. No food for breakfast.
- One tablespoonful of milk per day is allowed.
- Saccharin or Stevia may be used.
- No sodas of any kind
- No alcoholic beverages of any kind
- No diet teas
- No fruit juices or vegetable juices
- Some fruits and carbs are allowed
- Protein restricted to only chicken, white fish and lean beef
- Mixing vegetables is not allowed
- No exercise during phase two
- No medicines. Modern adaptations now allow for prescription medications.
- No cosmetics that contain any oils
- No lotions or topical creams
- No massages

<u>Sample Meal Plan</u>
BREAKFAST - Tea or black coffee
LUNCH - 100 grams of chicken breast, spinach, apple and one piece of melba toast
DINNER - 100 grams of flounder, cucumber slices, handful of strawberries, and one piece of melba toast
SNACK - None unless you save part of a meal to eat for snack later in the day.

There are many more detailed sample meal plans for the original protocol available on Pinterest and in some hCG cookbooks.

Dr. Simeons wrote, "I never allow any kind of massage during treatment. It is entirely unnecessary and merely disturbs a very delicate process which is going on in the tissues. Few indeed are the masseurs and masseuses who can resist the temptation to knead and hammer abnormal fat deposits. In the course of rapid reduction, it is sometimes possible to pick up a fold of skin which has not yet had time to adjust itself, as it always does under hCG, to the changed figure. This fold contains its normal subcutaneous fat and may be almost an inch thick. It is one of the main objects of the hCG treatment to keep that fat there. Patients and their masseurs do not always understand this and give this fat a working over. I have seen such patients who were as black and blue as if they had received a sound thrashing."

Chapter 11 - 2.0 Protocol

Dr. Zach LaBoube outlined phase two of the 2.0 protocol as follows:

- Daily protein calorie allowance is based of 40 percent of BMR
- Maximum daily carbohydrate limit is 30 grams. This can be either total carbs or net carbs.
- Eat breakfast
- No fruit
- No starches
- No sugars
- Continue supplements and prescription meds as advised by your physician
- Cosmetic use is allowed
- Use of lotions and topical creams is allowed
- Diet sodas and zero calorie drinks such as Crystal Light are allowed
- Protein is the central focus with many more options
- Unlimited mixing of vegetables within carb limit
- All calories counted come from a protein source
- Unlimited non-starchy vegetables allowed as long as you count the carbs
- Get 15 to 20 grams of protein within 30 minutes of starting your day
- Continue to exercise as you were doing prior to the diet, but do not add additional cardio beyond your regular routine
- Encourages 20-30 minutes of walking before breakfast

Sample Meal Plan
BREAKFAST - Coffee (with or without artificial sweetener), three egg white omelet with ½ cup spinach and ½ cup tomatoes
LUNCH - Tuna lettuce wrap with dill pickle relish and unlimited green vegetables
DINNER - 12 ounces of Mahi Mahi with broccoli
SNACK - Beef jerky (with zero carbs), one cup of chicken bouillon, ½ serving of whey protein shake

If you do not have time to cook during the day, you can substitute a whey or soy protein shake for a quick breakfast or lunch if you check the carbs and sugar listed in the nutritional label. Do not use any protein shakes that contain sugar as one of the ingredients.

Dr. LaBoube uses a formula referred to as P/FC, which means total protein in the food item divided by total fats plus total carbs. In his example, 3.5 ounces of chicken breast or 7 ounces of tilapia would have the same P/FC count. The P/FC essentially helps rank your protein and vegetables by what is healthiest for you in terms of weight loss. If I want to eat the biggest meal I can, I would choose a meal with all foods that have the highest P/FC rating. If I want a smaller meal, I can choose lower P/FC ranked foods in moderation. Foods with a P/FC rating of 4 or higher are going to be the recommended choices.

A protein chart for meats and vegetables in *HCG 2.0*. **These charts are not an approved food list. They are only in the book to demonstrate different P/FC calculations.** At this time, there is no approved food list for 2.0 because that list includes everything that does not contain sugar, fruit or starches. Obviously, some foods are much better for you to maintain a healthy diet than others. Even if they came out with a sugar free, carb free version of a Twinkie it would never equal the health benefits of whole foods.

According to Dr. LaBoube you do not need to count the calories from vegetables or from fats, if you are conscious of the carb count. The calories from fat should only be a by-product from your protein sources anyway. For me, it was easiest to record all of my foods, and then if I needed a little wiggle room at the end of the day I could subtract any calories I had added in from vegetables or fats. This was rarely an issue for me though. Too often I see people trying to decide whether to count a food as a protein or just the carbs. Make your life easier and record it all. It's a good habit to get into.

This part is important. The most common myths I find about the 2.0 protocol is that the only oils you can use are coconut oil or MCT oil, that you aren't allowed to eat dairy, the only sweetener allowed on the diet is Stevia, and that you can only eat low fat foods. Just to be clear, **this is not written anywhere in the book**. Those are all myths passed along within support groups because something caused one person to stall, or someone misinterpreted the book. None of these are true. It is true that in a blog post Dr. LaBoube stated that he believes dairy is empty calories, but he does not state anywhere that it is not allowed on the diet.

He does recommend using coconut oil and MCT oil, but he does not state that no other oils are allowed. He also recommends Stevia as the healthiest alternative to sweeten foods and drinks, but he does not prohibit other types of artificial sweetener. And he never sets a limit on fats. The book is written toward lower fat intake, but different bodies respond differently to fat, so he wisely leaves that up to each dieter to determine the fat intake that works best for their body. My recommendation is to start the first week or two with lower fat intake and then gradually increase your fats until you notice the point where it causes you to lose weight slower or stall.

If you are doing the hCG 2.0 diet it will be much harder to have a set meal plan because each dieter will have a different calorie limit within 500-800 calories, and those calorie limits will change for every 10 pounds lost during phase two. Many of you will experience big losses in your first week of the low-calorie diet. There is a convenient calorie calculator and P/FC calculator on our website at www.MyHCGWellness.net and on our mobile app My HCG Wellness available for free on iTunes and Google Play.

In a recent conversation, Dr. LaBoube told me, "My focus is on sustainable weight loss. I don't believe in providing dieters with menu and saying eat this. My philosophy is, 'give a man a fish and he eats for a day, but TEACH a man to fish and he eats for a lifetime.' My goal in writing the book was to teach people HOW to eat, not to provide them with a temporary menu change. I think this results in more sustainable weight loss. If people don't want to take the time to read the book, HCG 2.0 is probably not the diet for them."

So, how do you know what to eat without a meal plan? Much of that will depend on how frequently you like to eat. If you are like me, your breakfast routine is pretty much set in stone. I always have two hard boiled eggs and black coffee with an artificial sweetener. So, I know that my breakfast is 140 calories, 1.2 carbs, 10 grams of fat, and 12 grams of protein. When I pre-plan my meals for the rest of the day, I automatically subtract 140 calories and 1.2 carbs from my daily limit. For people who aren't creatures of morning habit, or for travelers, that doesn't always work since their breakfasts may vary.

Let's look at a few options for deciding how much to eat and when. You can divide your daily calories up by the number of meals you want to eat during the day. For example, if my limit is 600 calories per day I may want to eat 200 calories per meal. If I want a snack in the evening I may want to eat 150 calories for two of my meals, 200 calories for one meal, and 100 calories for a snack. However, some people may like to just graze throughout the day instead of eating meals at certain points throughout the day, so they may want to have six 100 calorie snacks instead of three meals. I know my preference often changes from day to day depending on the activities I have planned that day.

Most of the questions I see about the 2.0 diet are regarding how to know if they should count the calories in the food item as a protein, or to count the carbs. The easiest way I tell people to do this is to count everything. I use My Fitness Pal to record everything I eat or drink. As long as I stay within my carb and calorie limits, I am ok. I even allow myself plus or minus 100 calories and plus or minus 5 grams of carbs per day because I do count everything instead of just protein calories and vegetable carbs.

I spoke with a dieter this week who was really frustrated that her appetite still had not decreased and she hadn't lost weight after being on the drops for one week. When I asked her what she had been eating, she said she had just coffee for breakfast, a sandwich for lunch and steak and a salad for dinner.

Obviously, having a sandwich means you are consuming too many carbs per day, and many salad dressings have hidden sugars. And when questioned, she said she didn't even know what her calorie limits were. **So, let me stress this as much as I possibly can, taking hCG without following a diet will not give you the desired results. The weight loss comes from the diet.** It is up to you to read the published information on the protocol you choose for more detailed information before you begin taking the hCG. Know the diet guidelines.

Dr. LaBoube's website is www.InsideOutWellness.net.

Chapter 12 - 3.0 Protocol

For the chapter on the 3.0 protocol I have asked my friend Debbie O'Phelan to contribute, since she is one of the founders of the protocol. She has done a tremendous amount of research and has developed some great recipes that fit within the protocol. At the time of this writing, her book is still in the works, but you can find out more detailed information and even get personal coaching through her website at www.LoCarbCreations.com or her Facebook group called hCG 3.0 - Keto Assisted Weight Loss. Even without a book, she has changed the way I think about the hCG diet, and I have incorporated a lot of her ideas into the way I have dieted and even the way I maintain my losses. I feel it pushes the hCG diet even further from the original protocol than the 2.0 diet does, but still relies heavily on ketosis.

I believe this protocol takes a little more planning and work on the part of the dieter, but still has great results. And this is perfect for someone who really enjoys the foods with higher fat content and those who like a bigger variety of foods.

The following information in this chapter has been contributed by Debbie O'Phelan.

The 3.0 Keto Assisted Weight Loss protocol is as follows:
Fat loading in phase one is required, and it is recommended that you fat load for two days prior to the low calorie phase (phase two). Fat loading "clean" on healthy fats and keto foods are encouraged, this makes the transition to the low-calorie phase much easier and prevents a lot of weight gain. Most who load "clean" end up not gaining any weight, but actually losing weight instead.

Testing your fasting glucose is not necessary, but recommended. Once a person knows their average fasting glucose, it's easier to choose a protein amount that will make the ideal personalized conditions for weight loss.

Using the keto calculator in the file section of the hCG 3.0 Keto Assisted Weight Loss group on Facebook will personalize your macros based on the daily protein amount chosen. Calorie confusion will keep the body guessing what is next, so two sets of macros are chosen. One set of macros are at 40% deficit, the other set of macros set at 55% deficit. Each day these macros are cycled.

Tracking macros is very important as is getting as close as possible to your goals every day. My Fitness Pal Premium allows you to preset percentage deficits to your chosen macros so it automatically cycles your daily goals for you once you input the information. Tracking is essential. If you do not track your foods you will not do well on this program. Guessing just doesn't work.

Intermittent fasting is encouraged by either eating all your calories in a "window" of time or eating all your macros in one meal. At least 20 minutes of exercise is encouraged before the fast is broken. For example, if you like to walk or run or swim, do this before you eat your first meal of the day. This will give you the most impact and will increase your metabolic rate.

Food groups which are not part of the 3.0 keto plan are sugars, starches, grains and gluten. Some people may be able to eat berries in limited amounts.

You should continue all your current supplements and prescriptions. I recommend adding magnesium as well if it's not already part of your daily supplements, as well as electrolytes and sole water (water that has been fully saturated with natural salt) to keep blood pressure and blood glucose from dropping and to keep the "keto flu" at bay.

You can also continue your normal use of all cosmetics, lotions and oils.

Some zero calorie sweeteners are allowed. Research has shown some are better than others. The files section on the Facebook group 3.0 Keto Assisted Weight Loss lists these sweeteners.

A whole food approach is encouraged not only for weight loss but overall health as well. However, since we are all unique and our tastes and styles of eating vary, a person may choose to eat whatever they want daily if it fits into their personal macros, and avoids sugars, starches, and limits the carbs.

Fat fasts are used if a person stalls for three or more days or if weight loss has become sluggish. The file section in the Facebook group has suggestions on a variety of ways to do a fat fasts. The average loss during a fat fast is one pound per day, and it can be done for up to five consecutive days. Instructions for ending the fat fast are also in the files on the Facebook group.

You can stay on the hCG 3.0 Keto Assisted Weight Loss program if immunity doesn't set in. In the file section of the group we discuss how you can tell if you have developed an immunity to hCG. One member did the 3.0 Keto Assisted program for six consecutive months. She walked daily while fasting, practiced calorie confusion, fasted intermittently and used a fat fast when she stalled. She lost 70 pounds during that time before transitioning to phase three. Then she lost ten additional pounds in phase three and got down to her high school weight of 119 pounds. She has maintained those losses using the tools she learned in phase two.

You can continue to lose in phase three if you choose. In the file section of the Facebook group we have a file which discusses phase three and illustrates how to maintain weight loss or to continue to keep losing weight.

What I love about the hCG 3.0 Keto Assisted Weight Loss program is that it is tailor made for you as an individual. It's not a cookie cutter program because we are not all the same. From my own research and testing I have found not everyone does well eating a lot of protein, and not all do well eating fruit. Some people do better eating quite a bit of fat. I have found that your glucose readings will help determine your optimal macros for you individually.

I learned all of this based on my own struggles with various hCG programs and with having higher glucose. I could not figure out why I lost slow on other programs, why I could not maintain in phase three, and why I would gain the weight back only to repeat the cycle. I also was cold, lost hair and craved fat. My first clue was when I noticed the degree to which different keto groups varied in suggested protein amounts. Some were high protein low fat, others were high fat low protein, but I noticed not everyone did well in both groups.

My next clue came when I was researching intermittent fasting. I learned that protein, while very low on the glycemic index, is very insulinogenic. This means that in some people too much protein produces an excess of insulin in the body (especially those who suffer from insulin resistance). Too much insulin in the body gets stored as fat.

Everything was making sense to me. People with good or normal glucose need more protein to lose weight properly. People with higher glucose need lower protein to lose weight properly, and people with slightly elevated protein fall in-between and need an average protein between the two.

The hCG 3.0 Keto Assisted Weight Loss program was born from realizing that for a person to optimize their weight loss they need to choose the right amount of protein for their body, not just what is good for everyone else. Adding the benefits of intermittent fasting and calorie confusion with fat fasting just increases the impact of this hCG program and produces greater weight loss results. The average weight loss in a 23-day round is 17 pounds, and you never feel like you are deprived or "dieting".

Food choices are endless so they include everything you can fit within your daily macros while avoiding sugar, grain, glutens and starches. This includes anything from homemade ice cream, keto breads, keto pizza, keto burger and sandwich buns, keto Pad Thai, keto clam chowder, etc. I could go on and on about your choices. In the files on the Facebook group I have lots of menu suggestions and provide a 3.0 keto assisted recipe bundle with phase two through maintenance foods such as pizza crust, burger/sandwich buns, muffins, granola, monkey bread, tortillas and similar approved recipes.

A member who had never done the hCG 3.0 Keto Assisted Weight Loss program allowed herself to be tested using a Dexa fat percent scan before and after phase two. The recorded results are stunning. The weight she lost was 99% pure fat. This showed that almost all the weight she lost was pure fat on the 3.0 plan. She also noticed quite a few improvements on how she felt during the round. She didn't experience any hair loss, didn't experience cravings, and didn't feel the need to cheat. She said she did not feel as if she was dieting at all.

Here is an example of what a day looks like on hCG 3.0 Keto Assisted Weight Loss program for a 5'10 woman 54 years old weighing 220 lbs. Her macros would be:

- Her high calorie day with a 40% calorie deficit are 1021 calories, 78 fat grams, 60 protein grams, and 20 net carbs. She eats one meal a day or eats within a time window. She tracks and eats what she chooses to get as close to her macro goals as possible. She avoids sugar, starch, grains and gluten. She may have berries if it does not affect weight loss.
- Her next day she practices calorie confusion, so this day is a low-calorie day for her at 55% calorie deficit. This would be 766 calories, 50 fat grams, 60 grams of protein, and 20 net carbs.
- She cycles these days to confuse the body throughout the diet.

I provide one on one personal coaching on this program for a small fee. This coaching can be for phase two, phase three, or both.

Sometimes a person just needs daily accountability. All the members I have coached have learned lifelong skills on how to live their life making better eating choices on or off hCG. One member recently told me when she traveled she used being away from home as an excuse to eat off plan. But while I was coaching her she had the confidence to choose wisely and still enjoy herself. This had never happened for her before coaching. She came back from a mini vacation early in phase three with a weight loss of over two pounds.

Knowledge and confidence gives us the power to avoid future weight loss struggles. Some of the people I have coached have told me they may never need hCG again. I consider this a success. My goal with this program is to teach people not just how to eat while on hCG, but to use these same tools to keep their weight in check for a lifetime.

For more information on 3.0 protocol, visit Debbie's website at www.LoCarbCreations.com and her Facebook group called HCG 3.0 – Keto Assisted Weight Loss.

Chapter 13 - Rogue Dieters

Rogue dieting is when you make your own rules and vary your protocols from how they are originally written. Mention going rogue in one of the social media groups for any of the protocols, and you may likely find yourself kicked out of that group. Sometimes because the administrator for the group is extremely strict about protocol, but sometimes because they just do not want your post to confuse new dieters who are trying to find out about the protocol. Fortunately, there are also social media groups for rogue dieters where you can exchange ideas without condemnation.

The number one reason I see dieters fail on the hCG diet is because they start their first round with the intent of doing the diet their way instead of following a protocol. Then they give up after a week or two because they aren't seeing progress. It's not uncommon to hear someone say that they are going to keep eating the foods they normally eat but just cut back on calories. Or they are going to incorporate the hCG into their South Beach Diet or Mediterranean Diet. Those are usually the people who end up bad mouthing hCG and claiming it doesn't work.

I am all for going rogue on your hCG diet and customizing the diet to fit your lifestyle. I believe that is actually the best way to make long term changes in your diet. However, I strongly recommend that for your first round, and especially the first two or three weeks, that you choose a protocol and stick to it. The only time I recommend starting off-protocol is if your physician has customized the diet to meet your specific health needs. Fully commit yourself to doing the protocol exactly as written. Do not be that person who tries to see how far they can push the limits and still get away with it. If you do that I can almost guarantee you will only lose a fraction of the weight you would lose by focusing on excelling within the guidelines.

Do your best to stay focused on the guidelines and applying them one hundred percent. Then slowly begin adding in one food at a time to monitor how it affects your weight loss and digestive system. By starting with one of the tried and true protocols you will begin to see what your average daily losses will be. Granted, you may stall a time or two, but you will start to see if you average losses of a half-pound a day or a pound a day, etc. Then if you start to add in a food, such as peanut butter or cheese, you can see if that is a food that causes your weight loss to stall. And, because you have been abstaining from that food so far in your diet, you may even notice a food allergy by way of swelling, or upset stomach that you never noticed when that food was a part of your everyday diet.

Your rogue protocol may end up looking like a combination of all three protocols. I find that I am most successful in losing and feeling satisfied when I do the 2.0 protocol, but I incorporate a little higher fat and intermittent fasting. I do not add as much fat as in the 3.0 protocol or do the calorie cycling, but I consider it a combination between the 2.0 protocol and 3.0. And with the changes I have made I have found it easier to transition into a lifestyle way of eating by just raising my calorie limits and adding a few fruits in phases three and four.

Sometimes going rogue may look like going above or below the recommended calories, carbs or proteins as part of your daily routine, adding lotions or oils in the original protocol, or eating nothing but proteins one day per week. There are any number of variations you can make to any of the protocols, so it would be impossible to list them all here.

In summary, going rogue can be a very good thing in customizing your diet to work with your individual body. But unless you are using a protocol customized for you by your physician, I highly recommend starting with one of the three protocols mentioned earlier in this book for at least the first two or three weeks of your first round, and then make changes slowly and track your results to see if those changes work for you on the diet.

Chapter 14 - Intermittent Fasting

The clear leader right now on the subject of intermittent fasting is Dr. Jason Fung. He has two great books that I highly recommend. One is *The Obesity Code*, and the other is *The Complete Guide To Fasting*. Both books are available on Amazon or at your local bookstore. Dr. Fung stresses the effect of insulin on weight loss and how intermittent fasting can control your insulin levels. But there are so many other health benefits including detoxifying the body, lowering cholesterol, lowering the risk of type two diabetes, reduce inflammation in the body, triggers autophagy which can help shrink excess skin from weight loss, improve brain health, reduce the risk of cancer and reduce the side effects of chemotherapy, prevent Alzheimer's, and extend your lifespan. You can find much more detailed information in Dr. Fung's books.

The reason I mention intermittent fasting while doing an hCG diet is because I find it to be a great tool for breaking stalls, and it is recommended in the 3.0 protocol. I also use intermittent fasting frequently in phase three and maintenance to control my weight and the health benefits.

Dr. Fung mentions a few different ways to do intermittent fasting, but because we are already on a low-calorie diet in phase two, I have found my greatest success in doing the 16:8 fast. This means I fast for 16 hours and then consume all my calories within the remaining 8 hours of the day. I'm a night owl, so I choose later hours than some people would to do my fast. I eat between noon and 8pm and fast the remaining hours with only zero calorie beverages such as water or herbal tea. During those eight hours that I am eating I make sure I get in all my calories and daily macros I'm trying to reach.

It is important to keep drinking water during your fasting hours to avoid dehydration. Getting plenty of water can also help avoid headaches and keep you distracted from thoughts about eating.

Depending on your schedule you may want to move your eight hours to start earlier in the day, or you may need to stretch it to ten hours and only fast for 14 hours. Even 14 hours helps improve your insulin levels. Again, do not make yourself miserable. If you need to work up to 18 hours gradually or fast for fewer hours that is ok.

I encourage you to speak with your doctor before you begin fasting so your doctor can monitor the results from your fasts and to let you know if you have a medication or medical condition that would require you to alter your fast.

Chapter 15 - Before Photos And Measurements

Start by taking photos. It's up to you how much or little clothing to wear, but you want something that will accurately reflect your current weight. It makes a big difference if you are wearing a parka in your before photo and a swimsuit in your after photo. I recommend taking photos from front, behind, side and a close up of your face and neck area. No one else needs to see these but you if you choose. But you will want to see proof of the physical changes at the end of the diet.

Next, it's time to take some measurements. So, get out your measuring tape and something to record your measurements on. To get an accurate reading make sure to do the following:
- Use a non-stretchable measuring tape.
- Make sure the tape measure is level around your body and parallel to the floor when you measure.
- Keep tape close to your skin without depressing it.

<u>How To Measure</u>

Bust - Measure all the way around your bust and back on the line of your nipples.

Chest - Measure directly under your breasts, as high up as possible.

Waist - Measure at the narrowest point width-wise, usually just above the navel.

Hips - Measure around the widest part of the hip bones.

Midway (Gut) - Measure midway between the widest part of your hips and your waist.

Thighs - Measure around fullest part of upper leg while standing.

Knees - Measure immediately above the knee.

Calves - Measure around fullest part.

Upper arm - Measure above your elbows, around fullest part.

Forearms - Measure below your elbows, around fullest part.

Do not get discouraged here. These numbers will serve as motivation later.

Chapter 16 - Phase One Loading

The loading phase is essentially the same no matter which protocol you choose. You will begin taking or injecting the hCG on the first day as prescribed. On day one and two on hCG (which are referred to as phase one) you will consume as much fat as you can eat throughout the day. Yes, this may cause you to gain a few pounds, but it will definitely be worth it.

Loading is a crucial step in the hCG diet. I highly encourage you not to skip phase one. I know the thought of gorging before a diet seems counterproductive, but it is extremely important in the hCG diet. It provides an immediate calorie reserve to sustain you during the first few days of the very low calorie phase. The sudden increase in fat consumption triggers the metabolism of fat. So, it actually jumpstarts your diet.

In *Pounds And Inches* Dr. Simeons says the following: "One cannot keep a patient comfortably on 500 calories unless his normal fat reserves are reasonably well stocked. It is for this reason that every case, even those that are actually gaining must eat to capacity of the most fattening food they can get down until they have had the third injection. It is a fundamental mistake to put a patient on 500 calories as soon as the injections are started, as it seems to take about three injections before abnormally deposited fat begins to circulate and thus become available."

You will probably gain between 1-4 pounds during loading. If you are retaining water that number could be even higher. Do not panic. This is normal, and it will come back off during the very low calorie phase.

Proper loading will also help prevent a "starvation" reaction from your body and spike the liver enzymes. When you load, your brain tells the liver to increase the production of enzymes to help break up all the fats you are consuming. Then while your brain and liver are putting their energy on dealing with all the fats you have consumed, you can sneak into the very low calorie phase without shocking them into starvation mode. By the time your brain and liver are ready to respond to what you are doing, you will have already started burning away at the fat stored in your body.

So, live it up during the loading phase and get your fill of fatty foods. Many people choose to start their loading days during holidays or special events, such as a Super Bowl party or a birthday party. This gives them the opportunity to celebrate with food.

There are two ways to load for the hCG diet. The regular way is to eat as much of everything you want regardless of sugar and carb count. This way was the most fun for me because I could pig out on chocolate, pasta, pizza and ice cream. This is the way Dr. Simeons recommended patients load in his original protocol.

The second way is what is called "clean loading". Clean loading is when you load by eating high fat foods with little or no sugar and carbs. Someone clean loading may choose to eat things such as salmon, avocado, nuts and cheeses. Many dieters choose to clean load before they begin a second or third round since their bodies are no longer accustomed to high sugar and carb intake. For me, now that I have the sugar and carbs out of my system, if I eat too much of them now I feel bloated, nauseous or get a headache. Also, as a diabetic, clean loading helped prevent the spikes in my blood sugar.

<u>Sample Loading Menu</u>
BREAKFAST: 3 eggs, salmon, toast with peanut butter, real butter or cream cheese
LUNCH: cheeseburger, mayonnaise, avocado and chili-cheese fries, heavy on the chili and cheese
DINNER: salmon or tuna steak, loaded baked potato, butter, cheese, sour cream, veggies of your choice with melted cheese

SNACKS: nuts (cashews are the best for loading), chips, guacamole, celery, peanut butter, canned tuna, and avocado slices

A clean loading menu would not include the toast, buns, fries, potato, but may include things like pork rinds or bacon. Either way you load should be very enjoyable. My suggestion is to choose your way based on the types of foods you currently eat most.

The biggest thing to remember while loading is to eat fatty foods frequently throughout the day. You should feel full at all times. By the end of day two you will be begging to start the low-calorie phase.

Chapter 17 - Meal Prep

I have found the easiest way for me preplan my foods is to cook in bulk and divide up individual portions to freeze and thaw them as I need them. An example in 2.0 protocol would be to bake a few pounds of skinless chicken breasts, cut it up into bite sized pieces, divide it up into 100 gram servings and freeze each serving in a sealable sandwich bag. I label each bag with the content, calorie and carb info so I can pull out what I want to eat the night before and budget my calorie and carb content for the next day.

Each bag of chicken would be 165 calories and zero carbs. If I add to that a frozen bag of one cup boiled spinach at 41 calories and 6.8 carbs, I have a ready-made meal that is 206 calories and seven carbs. So, for dinner let's thaw out 100 grams of pre-baked cod fish (80 calories, zero carbs), one cup of steamed broccoli (50 calories, 10g carbs). If I add those to my two hard boiled eggs and coffee that I had for breakfast (I boil a dozen at a time), then I am only at 476 calories and 18g carbs for the day. So, I can have two cups of sugar free Jell-O and an ounce of sugar free beef jerky as snacks during the day. That puts me at 604 calories and 18g carbs in total.

Let's look at another example with a 700 calorie per day limit. If you do not like eggs for breakfast, you can try two slices of deli turkey breast (120 calories, 2 carbs) and one cup of cucumber slices (32 calories, 8 carbs). For lunch let's try 15 baked shrimp (120 calories, zero carbs), ⅓ head of lettuce (23 calories, zero carbs), one cup of cherry tomatoes (28 calories, 4 carbs), four tablespoons of Walden Farms Sugar Free Ranch Dressing (70 calories, zero carbs). For dinner, you may eat a three-ounce hamburger patty (113 calories, zero carbs) with one cup of mashed cauliflower (142 calories, 8.9 carbs). That puts you at 648 calories and 23 carbs with your meals, so you can add in six black olives as a snack (54 calories, 6 carbs). The daily total is 702 calories and 29 carbs.

These examples were just some ideas for quick and easy foods if you are like me and do not like to cook. If you do like to cook and want to try some of your favorite recipes or some of the hCG recipes, I suggest creating the recipe in your My Fitness Pal app to calculate your calories and carbs per serving before dividing it up to freeze so you can label them properly. Once you save the recipe in your recipe section of the app it will be available to you each time you eat it.

Make this a budgeting game or a puzzle to figure out which of your favorite approved foods can fit into your daily meal plan and plan ahead. Buy all of your ingredients and cook in bulk when you can. There are very few foods you can grab at the quick stop if you are in too big of a rush to eat, so do not wait until the last minute.

Chapter 18 - Traveling And Eating Out

Dieting on the road is rarely an easy task. The hCG Diet is no exception. Sometimes it is easier to have small snacks throughout the day, and sometimes your only option is to wait until mealtimes. And, if you are staying with friends or family, rather than in a hotel, you may feel obligated to eat whatever they are cooking. I will give you a few tips to incorporate as you can in whatever situation you are in.

1. Keep drinking as much water as you can. Stock up on bottled water, or better yet a refillable bottle. If it's helpful, keep water flavoring or herbal tea bags and stevia with you to add to your water. Just keep drinking it.

2. Bring a small ice chest with you, especially if you aren't staying somewhere that you have access to a refrigerator. Fill it with things like hard boiled eggs, carrot and celery sticks, and almonds. If you are doing 3.0 you can add cheese stick, peanut butter or containers of bacon.

3. Opt for the salad bar whenever possible, but be wary of the salad dressings. I often bring my own whenever I can. Many large grocery stores even have great salad bars available. Know your protocol well enough to know which items to avoid regardless of how tempting they look.

4. At hotel breakfasts and restaurants, opt for scrambled or hard boiled eggs whenever possible. Or for 3.0 choose sugar free yogurt, bacon and sausage.

5. Bring your own sweetener packets or drops. I'm often surprised how many places do not have any artificial sweeteners, especially when traveling outside North America.

6. If staying with family or friends, contact them ahead of time to let them know that you are on a strict diet, and even though you would most likely enjoy every meal they cook, that you would like to prepare your own foods, or better yet, offer to cook for your hosts. I love having overnight guests, but trying to guess what kinds of foods they will like often stresses me out, so whenever someone offers to supply their own food it takes a lot of pressure off of me. So, if necessary, stop at the grocery store on the way to their home to pick up a few essentials. But do not be surprised if they want to join you in whatever you are eating, especially if there are children there.

7. Bring a shaker bottle and protein powder to mix up a quick meal on the go.

8. If it's a holiday or special event and you feel like there is just no way to get out of cheating on your diet, make it a cheat meal, not a cheat day. Trust me when I say that adding foods back into your diet too quickly, particularly sugar and carbs, will make you feel ill, and you may end up spending more time in the restroom than anywhere else. So, follow up any cheats with extra water to try to flush the sugar and carbs out quickly.

9. Many chain restaurants have the nutritional information of their foods online. Do your research before you go to find out what your options are.

10. Ask the waiter for healthy options that work within your diet. Many places are used to special requests and do not mind working with you. Do not rely on the waiter to know the sugar and carb contents or all of the ingredients for every item on the menu.

11. Ask the waiter to hold the bread. Bread baskets are so darn tempting, but you can also ask them to bring you a burger or grilled chicken sandwich without the bun.

12. Ask the waiter to bring only half your meal and to bring the rest in a doggy bag for later.

13. Order off the kid's menu or appetizer list for smaller portions. Or better yet just an order of steamed vegetables of the side items menu.

14. If you aren't preparing the food yourself, you aren't reading the labels of all the ingredients to make sure of the sugar and carb content, so allow yourself some wiggle room. On days that you eat out, try to stay under on your carb count.

15. Remember, it's your diet and your body. Do not let yourself to feel pressured to eat or drink anything you do not want. You are responsible for your choices.

16. Dieters on the 3.0 protocol may have the upper hand while traveling if they are used to intermittent fasting, but this can be done on any of the protocols. If necessary, you can eat all or most of your calories and protein in one meal so you do not have to worry about finding diet friendly food but once per day. However, if you are diabetic, not used to intermittent fasting, or you will be exerting extra energy during the day with walking or standing, then make sure you keep a few healthy snacks with you in case you need them.

17. Always choose grilled or baked food over fried food.

18. We live on the ocean, so there are lots of days when we are on the water and I only have what's in my ice chest. So, I freeze a couple water bottles ahead of time to drink after they thaw and keep the contents of my ice chest cold. I also keep a small container of baked chicken already cut into bite sized pieces, a couple hard boiled eggs, a bag of carrots or

cucumbers and a small container of deli meats. This way I can graze on the food throughout the day as I get hungry without feeling like I have to be seated at a table eating a meal.

19. If you must have something sweet, carry individual servings of sugar free Jell-O with you.

20. Be careful with condiments. Skip them when you can.

21. Choose whole foods over processed foods whenever possible.

22. If you have been sitting on a plane or car for a long time, take a walk once or twice around the block or get on the treadmill at a leisurely pace for a half hour. Sometimes just a little exercise can stave off food cravings.

23. Buy a small travel size scale to monitor changes in your weight if you will be gone for a few days. NewlineNY makes a small travel size scale perfect for fitting in your suitcase that only weighs 20 ounces.

24. If a travel scale is not possible, pack a measuring tape or a pair of snug fitting pants or shorts that you can wear around your room. Whenever you notice them starting to get too snug or you notice the inches increasing, then you are either bloated or have put on a couple pounds. Time to re-evaluate your eating strategy.

If you have any other great tips for traveling or dining out, I would love to hear them. Please drop me a line on our website at www.MyHCGWellness.net, or send me a message on Facebook.

Chapter 19 - Protein Shakes, Green Smoothies And Juicing

I get a lot of questions about protein shakes and juicing while on the hCG diet, so it's definitely worth discussing.

Let's start with juicing. Currently there is little or no research about juicing while on phase two of the hCG diet. In the original protocol, you are not allowed to mix vegetables like you are in 2.0 and 3.0, so your juices would be pretty limited. My opinion on the subject is that if you would like to juice vegetables to add as a supplement to a meal or in a soup, that would be safe, but I cannot recommend juicing as a meal replacement in phase two. However, I am a big fan of juicing overall, especially in phase three or maintenance.

Protein shakes and green smoothies are a different story. Many people use protein shakes during phase two, but you must read the labels carefully. Look for protein powders that have no sugar, and are low on carbs and calories. And definitely look at the serving size. My husband recently purchased a protein powder that looked like it met the calorie and carb requirements he wanted, but the serving size was for only one half cup shake. That wouldn't be very filling.

Green vegetable smoothies are another great way to get all the nutrients of fresh vegetables without eating salad or cooking them with every meal. And by using the veggies raw, you are getting even more nutrients than from cooking them. My husband has trouble sometimes with the texture of some fruits and vegetables, but when they are used in a smoothie texture is not an issue. So, if you want to throw some leafy greens like spinach, kale, or lettuce with some water and cucumbers or avocado into a blender that is great. You can add in coconut oil, or if you are doing the original protocol add an apple or berries. Experiment by adding fresh ginger or unsweetened almond milk, moringa powder, turmeric, or even some of your favorite protein powder. You can easily find some great recipes online that you can customize to fit whichever protocol you are doing.

My recommendation for a protein powder that fits safely within the hCG requirements regardless of which protocol you are on is the Jay Robb Egg White Protein Powder. Each serving is 24 grams of protein, zero fat, zero sugar and only four carbs. I love to add in a little powdered no sugar peanut butter or unsweetened cocoa powder with a few drops of stevia for a sweet treat.

Another great option is the Jay Robb Whey Protein Isolate Powder with 25 grams of protein, zero fat, zero sugar and only one carb per serving. There are many great protein shakes available if you do your research. For more protein shake options, please see our website at www.MyHCGWellness.net. Please choose appropriately for whichever phase of the diet you are in.

I always make my shakes with water during phase two, but I like to mix it up by adding cocoa powder, flavored stevia, water flavorings such as Crystal Light, or powdered peanut butter (45 calories, 5 carbs and only one sugar per 2 tablespoons). Get creative if you can, just remember that fruit is not allowed on the 2.0 or 3.0 protocol. It is allowed on the original protocol.

Chapter 20 - Hunger

Let's talk about hunger. Most of the time during phase two, you shouldn't be hungry except for mealtimes. If you are used to overeating, you may be mistaking not being full with being hungry. So really take the time to think about if you really feel hungry, or if you are just not feeling full. This distinction will gradually become more pronounced as your metabolism resets itself.

If you skipped the loading days, you will feel hungry. Loading up on those fats is really important to avoiding the hunger in week one. This is why no hCG website or doctor will tell you to skip the loading phase.

Is this round three or four for you? If so, you may have developed a slight immunity to the hCG. After your second round Dr. LaBoube recommends waiting 6-8 weeks before starting another round to prevent immunity and avoid hunger in phase two.

If you are still experiencing hunger we can look at a couple options. First, make sure you are using the correct dosage. If you are using the Inside Out Wellness drops from our website at www.MyHCGWellness.net, you should be taking .5 ml three times per day or .75 twice per day. If you are still feeling hungry after day seven, try decreasing the drops by one or two drops. Do not increase. Increasing the drops may make you feel hungrier.

Another option is to take full advantage of the unlimited veggies during phase two until your hunger starts to decrease. Nibble on cucumbers or celery throughout the day.

Option number three is to make sure you are drinking enough water. Staying fully hydrated can ease hunger pains and help you to keep your mind off eating.

Option four, do not wait so long between meals or snacks. If you find yourself feeling hungry often, try breaking up your meals into smaller portions and dividing them up throughout the day. This may be particularly helpful for people with blood sugar issues.

Option five, chicken bouillon is only 15-30 calories.

Option six, quality organic beef jerky. An ounce or two will do wonders to curb hunger.

Option seven, eat a pickle. A small to medium pickle has no fat and only one carb.

Option eight, brush your teeth. The minty flavor helps take away food cravings.

Not hungry enough to eat all your calories for the day? This happens to me a lot. So, I find myself searching for calories to eat before bedtime. As a general rule, you should not eat less than 500 calories per day unless recommended by your doctor. Your body still needs calories to function properly whether you are hungry or not, and not eating at least 500 calories may actually cause you to gain as your body reacts negatively to further calorie restrictions. Even if you aren't hungry, try to keep your daily calorie intake between 500 and the calorie maximum established in whichever protocol you have chosen.

Chapter 21 - Alcohol

Can I drink alcohol while on the hCG diet? None of the protocols prohibit alcohol consumption. However, Dr. Simeons advises that you may feel the effects of alcohol faster than you did before you began the diet. I do drink while on phase two of the diet, but not nearly as frequently as I would if I were not dieting. I try to limit myself to one or two drinks per week.

Keep in mind that many forms of alcohol contain a lot of sugar and calories. My preference is a vodka and club soda with lime. That is only 65 calories and .9 carbs. My next choice would be champagne at 78 calories and 1.6 carbs. A shot glass of Bacardi rum is 97 calories and zero carbs per ounce, but you need to be careful what you mix it with.

A Bacardi with a diet soda would not be a horrible option, but it uses a big chunk of your calories. You can see how quickly those calories could add up. On the other end of the scale, a light beer runs around 110 calories and 6.6 carbs, a glass of merlot at 122 calories with 3.7 carbs, and a glass of Yellow Tail chardonnay is a whopping 228 calories with 5 carbs.

Debbie O'Phelan of the 3.0 protocol claims that her testing shows that some hard liquor can lower a person's glucose while keeping them in ketosis. I do not have access to her research on that one. For the details on that you would need to contact Debbie or find information on her group page.

Chapter 22 - Stalls

You want to scream and throw your scale across the room. I get it. No one wants to diet and not see results. But before you get mad at the scale, let's look at a few reasons that stalls happen and possible ways to fix them.

Obviously, one major reason for stalls is cheating on the diet. One day of cheating enough to throw your body out of ketosis will take on average two days to get back into ketosis. So that's like three wasted days of dieting. So, the first thing to look at is whether or not you stayed on protocol with what you have eaten over the last three days.

The second reason is exercise. Remember, on a very low calorie diet increased exercise, especially cardio, can drain the few calories you are consuming before your body can absorb them. On a high calorie diet this is a good thing. But with a low calorie diet it can be dangerous. I currently live on an island, and when we go to town we walk most everywhere because we have a boat instead of a car. On those days when we do a lot more walking than usual I notice my weight loss stalls as opposed to days when I stay within my normal routine. On days when you know you will be exerting more physical energy you may want to increase your calories slightly and decrease the amount of physical exertion.

Reason number three is not a pleasant one, but when was the last time you had a bowel movement? Is it possible that you are a little backed up? Sometimes the days all run together for me, so I make a note in my food journal on the days I have bowel movements. If it has been longer than three days a little suppository intervention helps go a long way.

Have you been sick? Started or changed doses in a medication? If so, you may need to speak with your physician, or just give your body a little time to heal and adjust.

Once you have eliminated sugar and most carbs you may start to notice more easily how your body responds to different foods. I always recommend you make note of what you notice in your food diary and share it with your physician the next time you have an appointment.

Food intolerance is a big thing. When we were eating overly processed foods every day it's harder to notice, but it can have long lasting effects on your health. I love cabbage, and it's a very healthy food, but I have a food intolerance for it. Whenever I eat cabbage I either stall or gain a pound. Certain foods will cause inflammation within your body that may not affect others. This could be a certain vegetable or meat, dairy, eggs, nuts, grains or fruits. Sometimes it's more specific like a food dye, seasoning, preservative, or most commonly gluten.

Inflammation is a natural protective response from your immune system that you have eaten something it is having trouble processing. Not like getting food poisoning, but like eating something you may be allergic to or foods that our body just doesn't want or need. This is a big issue for people with arthritis or digestive problems. Try looking back in your food journal to see if there are certain foods that cause your weight to stall, or that may make you feel tired or give you headaches. If so, these foods should be probably be eliminated from your diet. Your body will thank you.

As for the artificial sweeteners, you will hear arguments as to whether they stall your weight loss or they have no effect. For me they did not cause me to stall or slow my losses, and I wouldn't have made it through phase two without them. None of the versions of the diet discourages their use, but they do recommend using Stevia over the pink or blue packets you may normally use.

Dr. Simeons wrote, "After the fourth or fifth day of dieting the daily loss of weight begins to decrease to one pound or somewhat less per day, and there is a smaller urinary output. Men often continue to lose regularly at that rate, but women are more irregular in spite of faultless dieting. There may be no drop at all for two or three days and then a sudden loss which reestablishes the normal average. These fluctuations are entirely due to variations in the retention and elimination of water, which are more marked in women than in men.

The weight registered by the scale is determined by two processes not necessarily synchronized. Under the influence of hCG, fat is being extracted from the cells, in which it is stored in the fatty tissue. When these cells are empty and therefore serve no purpose, the body breaks down the cellular structure and absorbs it. However, breaking up of useless cells, connective tissue, blood vessels, etc., may lag behind the process of fat-extraction. When this happens, the body appears to replace some of the extracted fat with water which is retained for this purpose.

As water is heavier than fat the scales may show no loss of weight, although sufficient fat has actually been consumed to make up for the deficit in the 500-calorie diet. When such tissue is finally broken down, the water is liberated and there is a sudden flood of urine and a marked loss of weight. This simple interpretation of what is really an extremely complex mechanism is the one we give those patients who want to know why it is that on certain days they do not lose, though they have committed no dietary error."

Diuretics should never be used for reducing during phase two of the diet regardless of which protocol you have chosen.

So, do not panic if your weight is not dropping as fast as you wanted yet. Sometimes these things take a little time for your body to adjust.

So, what happens if you keep seeing stalls in your weight loss in P2? I'm going to address this early in P2 because I start getting questions from concerned dieters all throughout P2, and it will affect everyone at some point. Some answers are obvious. If you need to eliminate certain foods, then do it. If you are cheating on the diet, stop. If you aren't drinking enough water, drink it. If you need some quality time on the toilet, make it happen.

Dr. Simeons wrote, "A plateau lasts 4-6 days and frequently occurs during the second half of a full course, particularly in patients that have been doing well and whose overall average of nearly a pound per effective injection has been maintained. Those who are losing more than the average all have a plateau sooner or later. A plateau always corrects itself, but many patients who have become accustomed to a regular daily loss get unnecessarily worried and begin to fret. No amount of explanation convinces them that a plateau does not mean that they are no longer responding normally to treatment."

My personal recommendation for breaking a stall is intermittent fasting as discussed earlier in this book. But there are a few other options you can try if you choose not to fast.

In the original protocol, Dr. Simeons allows for an "apple day". An apple-day begins at lunch and continues until just before lunch of the following day. Dieters are permitted to eat up to six large apples per day whenever they feel the desire. During an apple-day no other food or liquids except plain water are allowed. They may drink just enough water to quench an uncomfortable thirst if eating an apple still leaves them thirsty. Most dieters feel no need for water and are quite happy with six apples. The apple-day produces a gratifying loss of weight on the following day, chiefly due to the elimination of water. This water is not regained when you resume your normal 500-calorie diet, and on the following days you should continue to lose weight satisfactorily.

However, since fruit is not allowed in the 2.0 protocol, Dr. LaBoube recommends drinking a Cali Kicker. Cali Kicker is a flashy name for a common detox protocol that has been around for years. It doesn't taste great, but you should see some loss of water weight and swelling.

The basic recipe for the Cali Kicker is:

>8oz warm water
>1 Tablespoon lemon juice
>1/8 teaspoon cayenne pepper
>1/2 Stevia pack (optional)
>1 Tablespoon of apple cider vinegar (optional)

The Cali Kicker is approved for all protocols

In the 3.0 protocol, they recommend a fat fast or a steak and egg fast to break stalls. Again, for more information on those you can check with their Facebook group.

If the apple day or the Cali Kicker do not work well for you in breaking a stall, you may want to go back and look at some of the reasons mentioned earlier as to what is causing your stall and take the appropriate action to remedy the situation.

Chapter 23 - Dieting Tools

Make it a habit to record in your food diary any changes you may experience in the weight loss/gain or how you are feeling physically if you vary too far off your target calories or off protocol. Sometimes for me I need to increase my fat intake slightly when I stall before I start losing weight again. Sometimes increasing my calories by 50 helps. Or I may need to decrease my salt intake. Keeping the food diary helps me to look back at what I have been eating that may have caused me to stall or feel sluggish.

If you are using a mobile app with a food database, you may see multiple entries for the same food. For example, if I do a search for hard boiled eggs, I get multiple results. One entry tells me that one hardboiled egg has 63 calories, 4.2 grams of fat, 0.3 carbs and .2 sugars. Another entry says that hard boiled eggs are 78 calories each with 5 grams of fat, 0.6 carbs, and 0.6 sugars. In these instances, I like to err on the side of caution and choose the entry with the highest numbers.

For foods with nutrition labels on the packaging, compare the entry in the app to the product label. Sometimes the portion sizes or nutritional values on the label will differ in some of the entries in the app's database. Sometimes this is caused from different flavors of the same food containing different ingredients, different portion sizes based on the packaging, or perhaps someone simply made the entry in the create food section who was only concerned with including the calorie information but left out carbs, fats and sugar.

I have one other tip if you are using an app such as My Fitness Pal. For recipes that you prepare often it saves a lot of time and calculating to add them to the My Recipes section in your food diary. You can add recipes directly from certain websites, or you can enter the ingredients manually with specific brand names and then divide the nutritional information by the portion size. This will save in your app so that you do not have to re-enter the ingredients every time you use that recipe.

Chapter 24 - Phase 3 And Maintenance

Phase three (which begins three days after you have completed your hCG doses) is often overlooked in most hCG books, and is frequently feared as you near the end of phase two. Usually this is because dieters have been so happy with their rapid losses that they fear putting the weight back on once they raise their calorie limit.

Have no fear. Phase three is actually a good thing. It gives your body a chance to replenish itself in ways that it wasn't able to do while in phase two. In phase two your body is working hard using the fewer calories to provide nourishment and create energy. In phase three your body gets a chance to relax a little and put that energy elsewhere if it needs it. It also allows the hCG to completely leave your body and prevent immunity in any further rounds you may choose to do.

You can still lost weight in phase three. It won't happen as quickly, but it will still happen because your metabolism will be much more efficient, and you can still incorporate the good eating habits that you become used to in phase two.

The protocol for phase three does not differ much if any throughout the three protocols. They all promote the following:
- Eat only until you are no longer hungry. Do not eat until you are full.
- Keep reading nutrition labels before you even purchase food at the grocery store. Be aware of what you are eating.
- Restrict sugar and starches to rare occasions and in moderation. They are not now and will never be your friend. If you are wanting to maintain ketosis during phase three, I recommend making sure that your carbs plus sugar do not equal more than 50 grams per day.

- Track your weight every day. Anytime your weight goes above two pounds over your weight on your last dose of hCG, do a steak and apple day (as discussed later in this chapter).
- If your weight goes up a little one day, cut back a little on your calories the next day.
- Increase your calories gradually. A good rule is to add 200-300 calories per day until you reach your new calorie limit. It may be helpful to eat smaller portions throughout the day instead of in three meals.
- Your new calorie limit should be approximately 80% of your BMR if you want to continue to lose weight or up to 100% of your BMR to maintain your weight.
- Add in fruits and grains gradually and pay close attention to any food intolerances you may experience when you re-introduce them to your diet.
- If you have been doing the original or a low-fat version of the 2.0 protocol, introduce fats slowly back into your diet. And start with healthy fats, like avocado.
- Make note in your food journal of foods that may be causing weight gain any time you notice it.
- Keep drinking the same amount of water you were drinking in phase two. Increase that amount if you are increasing your exercise.

Websites like Pinterest have lots of great recipes for phase three. Do some research and find some foods that you love. This is the way you want to be eating for the rest of your life to maintain your losses.

The most commonly prescribed correction for any day you have gone two pounds or more over your last dosage weight is a steak and apple day. On that day, you would fast until dinner, and then eat a large (8-10 ounce) steak with an apple or tomato for dinner. No other food should be consumed during that day. And of course, drink plenty of water.

If you are a vegetarian then obviously, a steak day will not work for you. I have heard of a few alternatives to the steak or apple day, but the results may vary depending on your body. So, you may want to try whichever sounds best, and then make note in your food journal of your results.

- Protein day - Eat nothing but various types of proteins throughout the day. No fruits or vegetables.
- Egg day - Eat 9-12 eggs throughout the day. Drink only water.
- Yogurt day - Eat only plain sugar free Greek yogurt throughout the day.
- Intermittent Fasting - As discussed earlier in this book, eat only during an eight-hour period during the day. Only consume water or zero calorie beverages the remaining hours. Use caution if you have a medical condition that this may aggravate.

If you are doing a steak day or alternative more than once per week, you may want to re-evaluate your stabilization weight. So, you may want to do the steak day or alternative only with a five or six-pound difference rather than a two-pound difference.

Sometimes, overeating is not the problem causing your weight gain. Sometimes things like an injury or illness, stress or lack of sleep may cause a temporary gain. Exercise or excess sun exposure can also cause a lot of water retention.

For me, a change in medication also caused my weight to go up until my body could adjust to the new medication. Also, if you are exercising more in phase three, keep in mind that you may be gaining muscle weight. So, keep those things in mind before deciding to do steak days or stressing about a couple of pounds. Sometimes things will just work themselves out with a little time.

Chapter 25 - Time Between Rounds

Dr. Simeons wrote in *Pounds And Inches*, "After 40 daily injections it takes about six weeks before this so-called immunity is lost and hCG again becomes fully effective." He states the dieters should wait a minimum of six weeks between rounds. He further recommended that after the second round dieters should wait eight weeks, between the third and fourth rounds wait twelve weeks, between fourth and fifth round wait twenty weeks, and between the fifth and sixth round wait six months.

However, convincing someone to wait between rounds after they have seen rapid weight loss in their first round is often difficult. Dieters get excited when they see results and they often want to keep going. Right now, I am mostly hearing doctors recommend waiting a minimum of three weeks between rounds if you are doing drops, and six weeks for injections, while maintaining a healthy diet in phase three. It is important to stabilize your metabolism for a while.

If your body is showing signs of adrenal fatigue, your doctor may recommend you wait longer to start another round. I highly encourage everyone to wait at least the minimum three weeks and then really pay attention to whether you feel healthy enough to start your next round. If feel like you need longer between rounds or you know you have an event coming up that will interfere with you completing a successful round such as a surgery, wedding, guests staying with you or anything else that may interfere with your diet routine, then I advise you to wait longer.

There is no period too long to wait between rounds. So, it could be three weeks or three years. It is up to you if and when you do another round.

Chapter 26 - Naysayers And Critics

If you have questions or find the guidelines for any of the protocols confusing, please ask me or join any of the hCG Facebook groups to ask for support. Almost all of the members of those groups will happily answer questions. However, keep in mind that some groups follow the original protocol from *Pounds And Inches*, and some will follow the hCG 2.0 or 3.0 diet. Be conscious of the differences in the support groups and on recipe website. Remember the differences in protocols as discussed earlier in this book. And if you think you are getting faulty information from a group member, message the group administrator directly.

I have recently had disagreements with a group administrator on one group who was posting that artificial sweeteners are not allowed on the hCG 2.0 diet. As it turns out, she felt they stalled her weight loss, but they are allowed in the 2.0 protocol even though the recommended sweetener is Stevia. After I pointed this out she started posting that artificial sweeteners are not recommended, but she quit stating that they weren't allowed.

Some group administrators will want to push their own products on you claiming that theirs are better and that you cannot be in the group if you are not using one of their products. So just be conscious going in that some people will have their own agenda.

Be sure to read any group rules before posting to make sure they are using the same protocol you have chosen, and do not mention hCG brand names or product links unless that is allowed within that group.

Chapter 27 - Choosing Which Form Of hCG To Use

Unfortunately, I see people struggle with this question way more than I believe they should. You do have many great options that will give you similar results, and one option I definitely would avoid. Over the next few sections I will discuss the different options.

If you are getting your hCG through a weight loss clinic they will probably require that you use one of their products, so your options may be limited, but I recommend reading about each of the options in the next few sections just to help you decide which route to choose, especially if you are considering doing more than one round.

Prescriptions hCG

Prescription hCG can be ingested through injections, drops, sprays, pellets, or even a cream, but most doctors will prescribe it as injections. Legally in the United States you need a prescription from a doctor to obtain full strength hCG. Therefore, this is usually a more expensive option than some of the others, but you are more likely to get a real and consistent hCG product. For me, the biggest benefit of the injections is that you only have to remember to take the hCG once per day.

The drawbacks are the price, worrying about measuring exact amounts when mixing, and the occasional bruising from having to inject yourself. And if you are trying to buy hCG without a prescription you will not be able to purchase it from a reputable pharmacy which can ensure you are getting a quality product that contains real hCG from a healthy source.

Occasionally you will find a doctor that will allow you to take the prescription hCG orally through drops or pellets rather than as an injection, but the most common way is through injection.

Some of you will be lucky enough to find a compounding pharmacy or clinic that will pre-mix and fill your syringes for you. This usually comes at a higher price, but it is so much easier. All you need to do with these is to keep them in a dark spot in your refrigerator until you are ready to use them.

If you order your prescription hCG online you will most likely find that the company you order from will not sell the syringes. This can make ordering frustrating when everything is sold separately, especially if you are anxious to get started. To properly mix and use the prescription hCG you will need the vial of hCG, a bottle of bacteriostatic water, a mixing syringe and a separate injection syringe for each day as well an alcohol swab for each day.

There are numerous videos online about how to mix the hCG and how to give yourself the injections, so I won't go into all of that here, but I will recommend that you use 29 gauge 3 ml syringes with a ½ inch needle for your injections, and that you order enough for the complete round before beginning a round. Do not re-use or share syringes.

Some of the common brands you will notice are Hucog, Pregnyl, Novarel, Ovidrel, Corion, Fertigyn, and they will usually come in doses of 2,000iu, 5,000iu, or 10,000iu. The different dosage will determine how much bacteriostatic water you will need to use to dilute the hCG. When it comes to brands, I honestly cannot say that one specific brand works better than the others. They all work basically the same.

Most of the time you will receive a vial with the hCG in tablet form. You will need to inject bacteriostatic water into the vial to dissolve the hCG tablet before filling your syringes. This involves measuring your water to hCG ratio very carefully. Because of all these steps and measuring I find the injections to be more trouble, but I do get consistently good results with injections.

Once the hCG has been mixed with the bacteriostatic water it will be good for three to four weeks. So, if you are doing a long round, you will need to mix a new batch before your round is finished.

Homeopathic Drops

The next option, and the one I prefer is the homeopathic drops. These are much easier in that everything is already mixed for you, and you do not have to inject yourself. I have found that I get the exact same results that I got with the prescription injections as long as I chose I quality brand of homeopathic drops. These usually do not require refrigeration as long as you keep them out of heat and direct sunlight. So, they are ok at room temperature, which makes it much more convenient if you take them in your purse or suitcase when traveling.

Homeopathy is a natural system of healthcare that involves minimal dosage or micro-dosing. And with hCG you will get the most results with the least amount of hCG. So, when you look at a bottle of hCG you may see something that looks like this listed in the ingredients on the label: hCG 6x, 12x, 30x, 60x

The numbers refer to the number of times the original hCG substance was micro-diluted and succussed. According to homeopathic principles, each level of dilution has a different electromagnetic energy signature, which interacts with the various cells in the body differently. The higher the number, the more times the hCG has been diluted and put through the succession activation process. Therefore, by making a combination remedy that includes potencies of 6x, 12x, 30x, 60x, the remedy will have a slightly broader spectrum effect than one with just 30x.

Homeopathic drops should come with a vial to aid you in putting the drops in your mouth. It is recommended that you not eat or drink anything for at least 10-15 minutes before and after taking the drops so as not to prevent any absorption in the body. Depending on the brand, you would fill the dropper to the fill line before putting them under your tongue or you would count the drops as you put them under your tongue. I find it is hard to see the drops as I am putting them in my mouth without looking in the mirror, so I prefer drops with a dropper that has a fill line marked on it.

Let's use the Inside Out Wellness drops as an example when we talk about the frequency of dosing with homeopathic drops. With these drops you would take a total of 1.5 ml per day broken down into two or three doses. If you take the drops in the morning and at night only you would take .75 ml in each dose as indicated on the dropper. If you take the drops three times per day you would take .5 morning, mid-day and at night. You will get the same results either way because you are consuming the same amount each day. For that reason, it seems logical that only having to remember to take the drops twice per day instead of three times would be easier. However, if you know in advance you are prone to forget one of your doses during the day, you may choose to take the drops three times per day.

I have tried a few different brands of drops. I did not have great results with some of them even some people who say they love their results. The brand of drops that I consistently get great results from are the Inside Out Wellness drops, and they are made in an FDA approved pharmacy.

Non-Hormonal Drops

Despite what the advertisers may say, these are drops that do not contain hCG. They are strictly appetite suppressants, and therefore may have negative side effects if they even work at all.

At least once per week I hear someone making statements where they have confused homeopathic and non-hormonal hCG. I even see it on many websites about hCG. They are two different types of drops claiming to do the same thing. The big difference is that one contains hCG and the other does not. Non-hormonal drops can often be found at discount chain store and many places online.

Non-hormonal drops will also list many ingredients such as mango extract, L-Ornithine, L-Arginine, and L-Glutamine. While they may be useful ingredients in aiding weight loss, they still do not contain hCG. Keep in mind that anyone trying to sell you something is going to tell you that their brand is the best. Your best bet for finding non-prescription hCG is to find a reputable company that offers options, and do your research. Talk to people who have tried different products to find out what worked for them, and what was a waste of money or had negative side effects.

Do they work? Results vary greatly even within the same brands. This could be a placebo effect, or it could be that the ingredients work better for some people than others. The cost is not that much different from a quality homeopathic drop, so for the money I would recommend the homeopathic drops way before I would recommend non-hormonal.

Chapter 28 - Choosing A Start Date

Preplanning will really pay off when choosing a start date. As a general rule of thumb, you do not want to be in phase two for any special events or occasions when you know you will be eating a lot of food. So, you want to plan to start your diet to where you are in phase three or maintenance for your event, or wait to start until after your event. An example would be Thanksgiving dinner, or the wonderful buffet on a cruise ship. If you want to lose weight before the event, you will need to start your diet at least 45 days in advance for a long round, but preferably two months prior to your event so you have a chance to stabilize for a while in phase three.

The other option is to use your event as one of your loading days. Thanksgiving and the Friday after are perfect days to load because you can eat all you want on Thanksgiving and eat your fill of leftovers the next day.

If you do not need to plan around an event I always recommend doing your loading days over the weekend or two consecutive days when you won't be at work and can eat as much and as often as possible. It's very likely that at the end of each of your loading days you will feel bloated and uncomfortable. Then begin your low-calorie phase when you start back to work or on a day when you will be too busy to worry too much about food.

If you will be away from home, it's a good idea to carry extra snacks with you for at least the first two or three days just in case your body is still adjusting to the hCG and you find yourself feeling overly hungry. I recommend bringing things like cucumber slices or sugar free beef jerky. That way when you do feel hungry you will be less likely to head to the vending machine full of carb and sugar heavy snacks. Sometimes, just a little extra caffeine will help, so if you are a coffee drinker you may want to have an extra cup when you are feeling hungry.

Chapter 29 - Missed Doses

What if I miss a dose? One missed dose won't hurt you, but multiple consecutive missed doses will. The hCG should build up and stay in your system for three days, so after the first week you probably won't even notice one missed dose. Some people even skip one day a week when taking hCG injections.

If it has been less than four hours since your missed dose it won't hurt to take it late.

If you cannot remember if you took your dose, it is better to skip it. You may want to find a way to mark it on your calendar or in your notes section of My Fitness Pal with what time you took your doses to help you remember if you took them.

Chapter 30 - Cheat Days

What can I say here other than do not do it? One cheat day can kick you out of ketosis, which will take you approximately three days to get back into ketosis. So, one cheat day is like four wasted days of dieting. So really think about whether it will be worth it before you cheat.

A big reason so many of us gained weight to start with was our lack of self-control when it comes to food. So, make changes in your habits that will last a lifetime and stay the course.

If it's a birthday or anniversary or something where you really feel like you need to go off the diet, try to limit yourself to a cheat meal or snack instead of a whole cheat day. The fewer carbs and sugars you consume will make going back into ketosis much faster. If you are eating at someone's house who has prepared food especially for you without taking your diet into consideration then eat much smaller portions or just a bite or two of special dessert.

The best way to avoid cheats is to pre-plan. Eat before you leave the house whenever possible or bring your food with you. Do not wait until the last minute to think about your next meal or snack. Keep healthy foods in your kitchen and with you when you leave home whenever possible.

Chapter 31 - In Conclusion

I hope this book has been helpful in giving you more information on the hCG diet and helping you choose which protocol would work best with your lifestyle. Do not let the choices overwhelm you. If you choose a protocol that you feel is not working for you, you can easily change at any time. But most importantly listen to your body.

If you ever feel like something is not right, discuss it with your physician to see if what you are feeling is related to the diet or if something else is wrong.

Reach out for support whenever necessary. Remember that occasionally in support groups you will find advice that may not be within the specific protocol the way it was written. Not everyone that gives advice will be as well informed as others. So, if something doesn't sound right, keep asking around or better yet, go to the original source of the protocol.

On my website www.MyHCGWellness.net you can find more information on the hCG diet, a blog about my husband (A Man's Perspective) and my personal experiences with hCG, calculator tools, inspiring testimonials, and links to purchase quality hCG through both prescription sources and homeopathic drops. You can also contact me directly with questions or comments.

If you choose to do the 2.0 protocol, you can find the links to download our mobile app and our Facebook group for 2.0 recipes.

And please feel free to share your success stories and photos with us. We love to celebrate your victories. Here's to a thinner and healthier future. Let's tip the scales in your favor.

WWW.MYHCGWELLNESS.NET

Glossary

Terms and Acronyms

ACV - Apple Cider Vinegar

hCG - (Human chorionic gonadotropin) - A hormone produced by the placenta after implantation.

Hypothalamus - The area of the brain that secretes substances that influence pituitary and other gland function and is involved in the control of body temperature, hunger, thirst, and other processes that regulate body equilibrium.

Ketosis - The metabolic process that occurs when the body does not have enough glucose for energy. Stored fats are broken down for energy, resulting in a buildup of acids called ketones within the body. The aim of a ketogenic diet is to burn off unwanted fat by forcing the body to rely on burning fat for energy, rather than carbohydrates.

LDW - Last Dosage Weight

MCT Oil - (Medium Chain Triglyceride) - This is a tasteless oil that is considered a good source of energy that is easy for the body to metabolize. The name refers to the way the carbon atoms are arranged in their chemical structure. Sometimes MCTs are used along with medications for treating food absorption disorders including diarrhea, steatorrhea, celiac disease, liver disease, and digestion problems due to partial surgical removal of the stomach or the intestine. Athletes sometimes use MCTs for nutritional support during training, as well as for decreasing body fat and increasing lean muscle mass. MCT oil can be purchase in liquid form, and it occurs naturally in coconut oil.

P1D1 - You will see this often when people refer to which stage of the diet they are in. P stands for Phase, and D stands for day. P1, or phase one is the two days in which you load calories and fat.

P2 or phase two is the very low calorie phase.

P3 or phase three is after you finish the medication, you have increased your calorie intake to a suggested amount, but are still avoiding starches and sugar.

P4 or phase four is the stage in which you have gradually added some starches and sugar back into your diet. Phase four is also referred to as the maintenance phase.

PFC - Protein/Fats + Calories. By calculating the PFC on foods, you can rate your protein items. The higher the PFC number, the better the food is for achieving weight loss. If you want to eat a bigger meal, you would select a food with a higher PFC value.

POP - Perfect On Protocol - Following the diet exactly

R1 - Refers to round one or your first time doing the diet. If you restart the diet again after your first round that would be R2 and so on. This is often seen as R1P1D1, which would mean round one, phase one, day one.

Released - Another way of saying the amount of weight lost.

Stall - If you have stayed on protocol but have not lost any weight for a couple days, we refer to this as a stall.

Steak Day - In phase three, if you find your weight has increased by two pounds over your last dosage weight, a steak day is recommended.

VLCD - Very Low Calorie Day (or Very Low Calorie Diet)

Made in the USA
Lexington, KY
27 June 2018